Emotions &
Essential Oils

Also by Rebecca Linder Hintze:

Essentially Happy
Essential Oils for Happy Living
Healing Your Family History

Emotions & Essential Oils

An A to Z Guide

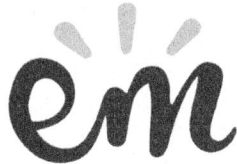

Rebecca Linder Hintze, M.Sc.

An Emotions Mentor™ Book

Visium Group,
LLC Leesburg, Virginia

The type for this book is Smoothy Sans.

Visium Group LLC
Leesburg, Virginia
www.rebeccahintze.com

Cover and interior design by Nick Hintze
Copy editing by Stephanie Gunning

978-0-9993301-2-8 (paperback)

Ordering Information:
Special discounts are available on quantity purchases by corporations, associations, and others. For details, contact the publisher at the website above.

CONTENTS

INTRODUCTION

The standard guidelines for emotional wellness include consumption of a nutritious diet (with supplementation whenever needed), elimination of unhealthy foods and other substances from your diet and environment, adequate water intake, proper sleep habits, exercise, a resourceful outlook on life, and choosing only to engage in respectful, supportive relationships. In addition, essential oils can have a positive emotional impact on you by elevating your mood, promoting relaxation, and contributing other healthbenefits.

In your hands, you are holding an A to Z guide to individual essential oils and common essential oil blends you can either purchase from a reputable essential oil producer or make yourself at home in the proportions of your own preference.

WHAT IS AN ESSENTIAL OIL?

Essential oils are concentrated liquids made from different parts of plants—everything from stems, leaves,and flower petals, to roots, seeds, needles, wood pulp, bark, and berries. Depending on the source material, harvesting and oil production may be handled in a few different ways, cold pressing or steam distillation are two examples. The resultant essential oil retains thechemical constituents of the plant, which are scented and may have a variety of therapeutic properties.

THREE WAYS TO USE ESSENTIAL OILS

Essential oils are used in three primary ways:

    1. **Aromatically,** smelled right out of the bottle or in a mist produced by a diffuser. Water diffusers are popular.

    2. **Topically,** either neat, if an oil is mild and labeled as "safe" by the manufacturer; or diluted in a carrier oil.

    3. **Internally,** if labeled as "safe for human consumption." *(Note: Essential oils are regulated by the U.S.*

Food and Drug Administration as nutritional supplements. Every nation has its own regulatory agencies and laws.)

For the management of your moods, as described in this book, I recommend using the essential oils aromatically and topically.

AROMATHERAPY

To gain the aromatic benefits of essential oils, try:

- Holding the bottle near your nose and inhaling Begin cautiously, as some undiluted oils have intense aromas.

- Pouring a couple of drops of an oil directly from the bottle into the palm of one hand, then rubbing both hands together, cupping your palms in front of your nose, and inhaling deeply for a few breaths.

- Filling a water diffuser with about a half cup of water and adding four drops of essential oil (or blended oils), and running it in the space where you are for a while.

- Putting a few drops of oil in steaming water, covering your head with a towel and breathing in the scent. This method is like visiting a steam bath.

APPLYING OIL ON THE SKIN

Oils have different properties. As a result, some, like marjoram and oregano, are warming. Some, like peppermint, are cooling. And they are warm or cool in varying intensities.

If you are unfamiliar with the properties of an essential oil, the best way to introduce it to your skin is in a diluted form. Think of dilution strategies as 4:1, 3:1, 2:1, and 1:1. This is as opposed to applying an undiluted oil *(neat application)*. If you ever feel that the intensity of an oil is too great, dilute further using a carrier oil that contains vegetable-based fats. *(Note: Essential oils themselves are not greasy.)*

Common unscented or lightly scented carrier oils are:

• Coconut oil.
• Fractionated coconut oil.
• Almond oil.
• Jojoba oil.
• Grapeseed oil.
• Olive oil.

Carrier oils are wonderful because, among other things, they help the essential oil to be spread over a larger surface area of the skin, and help the oil to linger in a local region of the body for longer without evaporating. Emotionally, the sensation of touch is soothing to the nervous system—even when you are smoothing an oil on your own skin it is comforting.

Massage done with essential oils is extra pleasurable because of the aroma, and depending on the essential oil or combination of essential oils that is used, the therapeutic benefits may be enhanced. This type of experience has both kinesthetic and aromatic benefits. Cypress oil, for example, is healing for sore muscles—bringing us the joy of relief.

WHY SCENT AFFECTS OUR EMOTIONS AND HEALTH

Human beings are animals—yes, we are! And recent science has revealed that our sense of smell is more astute than commonly believed. A May 2017 article in the New York Times explained that early twentiethcentury researchers downplayed the impact of scent on our lifestyle to make us feel superior. Effectively, they blocked us from exploring our birthright.

Several different parts of the brain are involved with the sense of smell, including centers of the brain that pertain to emotions, memory, and learning. Scent can attract or repel us—perhaps warning of danger or suggesting that a specific food may be good to eat. It can also help to stimulate us or sedate us—largely because the molecules of scent attach to receptor sites in brain cells that release neurotransmitters like dopamine, GABA, serotonin, and endorphin, which regulate our body chemistry and tens of thousands of physical functions.

Although scientific researchers are only just now starting to understand why scent affects us so powerfully, we have thousands of years of anecdotal knowledge to draw upon from traditional usage in cultures around the world. Plant medicine was the earliest form of medicine. Given advances in technology, it is only a matter of time before our understanding is complete.

Every thought and feeling has its own chemical signature, which affects one or another of our organ systems for better or for worse. We know, for example, that people who are angry and resentful are more prone to heart attacks than people who are grateful and forgiving. If we want to promote heart health using essential oils, then wouldn't it make sense to use oils that help to reduce anger and promote gratitude?

From the perspective of tradition, we can extrapolate that the essential oils that promote certain emotional states may produce recognizable health benefits within our bodies. Even so, let's never forget that aromatherapy is holistic—meaning, the entire body is impacted by anything we smell. Not just the nose. Not just the little toe on the left foot. The whole body.

Healthy people tend to be happier.
Happier people tend to be healthier overall.

ESSENTIAL OILS AND OUR NEUROTRANSMITTERS

Neurotransmitters are chemical messengers that carry signals between brain cells. One of the most important of these is **dopamine**, which is involved with many of our daily behaviors. According to Science News for Students, dopamine plays a role in motivation, memory, learning, feeling rewarded, and habits.

Essential oils that can stimulate the body to produce more dopamine include: clary sage, jasmine, lemon, patchouli, Roman chamomile, and rosemary. Some scientists say **serotonin** is a neurotransmitter, others say it is a hormone. Whichever it is, its presence is associated with mood, appetite, sleep, sexuality, and pleasure. According to Medical News Today, between 80 and 90 percent of serotonin is in the gastrointestinal tract. But the serotonin the brain uses must be produced within it. If we run short of serotonin, we may experience insomnia, depression, low libido, and aggression.

Essential oils that can stimulate the body to produce more serotonin include: clary sage, lavender, lemon, marjoram, oregano, Roman chamomile, rose, rosemary, and wild orange.

Important to our moods is **norepinephrine** (aka noradrenaline), which is associated with mental alertness, concentration, focus, and our stress responses. If we run in short supply, we may feel foggy, irritable, and anxious.

Essential oils that can stimulate the body to produce more noradrenaline include: black pepper, grapefruit, lemongrass, and rosemary.

Acetylcholine was the first neurotransmitter to be discovered and it has both excitatory and inhibitory functions. In the central nervous system, it is excitatory: "It plays a role in arousal, memory, learning, and neuroplasticity. It also helps to engage sensory functions upon waking, helps people sustain focus, and acts as part of the brain's reward system." In the peripheral nervous system, its helps with contractions of cardiac, skeletal, and smooth muscles. Imbalances of acetylcholine may lead to fatigue. They can also be perceived in people with both Parkinson's disease and Alzheimer's disease, although for different reasons.

Essential oils that can stimulate the body to produce more acetylcholine include: lavender, lemon, rosemary, tangerine, wild orange, and ylang ylang.

The final neurotransmitters we will discuss are **glutamate** and **GABA** (gamma aminobutyric acid), which are sort of a pair. Glutamate encourages nerves to fire and send impulses. GABA tells nerves not to fire, so it calms the nervous system. Without enough GABA, our moods can become severe: We may get irritable, anxious, jittery, panicked, or even experience seizures (as a worst-case scenario). Caffeine inhibits the release of GABA.

Essential oils that can stimulate the production of GABA include: bergamot, clary sage, geranium, lavender, lemon, rose, sandalwood, and wild orange.

According to SelfHacked.com, the brain needs glutamate to form memories and engage in thinking. Imbalances are linked to major disorders, which include autism, epilepsy, schizophrenia, and depression, as well as neurodegenerative conditions like Alzheimer's disease, multiple sclerosis, and ALS (aka Lou Gehrig's disease).

Essential oils that can stimulate the body to produce more glutamate include bergamot and lavender.

HOW TO SELECT AN ESSENTIAL OIL

No matter what is going on in our head space and heart at any given time, essential oils can enhance our emotional state. Emotions are energy in motion, and we are most healthy when we acknowledge them and allow them to flow through us without getting stuck in us, without us getting attached to them, and without repressing them.

Negative emotional states, like apathy, anger, guilt, fear, sadness, irritation, and worry, are stressful.

Positive emotional states, like calmness, contentment, trust, joy, excitement, and passion, reduce stress.

In general, positive emotional states are more healthful than negative states. But we should always remember that emotions—all sorts of emotions—are a natural aspect of life in a human body. They give us valuable information about where we are, what's working or not working for us, and what actions we need to take to resolve our issues (whether physical, mental, emotional, or spiritual) and reestablish harmony, equilibrium, and composure.

For instance, the sadness of mourning a loss can feel smothering if we get stuck in it. But in the short term it reminds us of how much love we feel. We can anticipate the relief of returning to a neutral state after feeling sad, and then having another, hopefully happier emotion.

The excitement of riding a roller-coaster or winning a contest, by contrast, feels exhilarating in the short term. But extended happiness can begin to feel manic and tire us out. Even with positive emotions, we can look forward to the calm that comes after we regain our inner balance.

Essential oils can aid our naturally cycling emotional process when we use them to enhance and/ or shift how we feel at any given moment. Everybody reacts to oils in their own manner; be aware that it is important to play with the oils to discover your personal preferences and observe how your individual body chemistry is affected. As you become familiar with what works for you, your selections will be more intuitive.

POSITIVE EMOTIONS AND OILS THAT CAN PROMOTE THEM

Use the list below to begin a journey of emotional exploration.

Compassion/empathy. Compassion and empathy support the heart and lungs and promote flexibility, circulation, and overall wellness.
Essential oils: frankincense, lime, patchouli, rosemary, and the Comforting blend.

Courage. Courage strengthens the structural system (bones, muscles, ligaments), the respiratory system, the immune system, and mental performance.
Essential oils: arborvitae, cinnamon, clove, thyme, white fir, and the Uplifting blend.

Gratitude. Gratitude supports the heart, promotes hormonal balance and sleep, and reduces inflammation.

Essential oils: cypress, jasmine, rose, tangerine, and the Inspiring blend.

Joy. Joy and a sense of abundance or expansiveness boost the immune system.
Essential oils: cinnamon, frankincense, ginger, petitgrain, wild orange, and the Uplifting blend.

Love/trust. Love and trust support the heart, structural systems (bones, muscles, ligaments), the endocrine system, immune system, liver, gallbladder, and kidneys.
Essential oils: bergamot, geranium, juniper berry, lavender, and the Renewing blend.

Satisfaction/peace. Satisfaction and peace support brain functions like cognition, blood flow, and the endocrine system.
Essential oils: basil, coriander, melissa, peppermint, rosemary, the Metabolic blend, the Reassuring blend, and the Uplifting blend.

NEGATIVE EMOTIONS AND OILS THAT MAY HEAL THEM

Use the following list to explore ways to restore harmony.

Anger. Anger affects the liver and kidneys and may contribute to infections.
Essential oils: geranium, helichrysum, lemongrass, melaleuca, melissa, oregano, thyme, and the Renewing blend.

Anxiety/fear/terror. Anxiety, fear, and terror affect the brain, nervous system, heart, kidneys, and intestines.
Essential oils: basil, frankincense, lavender, peppermint, rosemary, vetiver, and the Reassuring blend.

Burdened. Feeling burdened affects the shoulders, upper spine, neck, and low back.
Essential oils: lemongrass, marjoram, white fir, the Grounding blend, and the Soothing blend.

Guilt/shame. Guilt and shame affect the stomach, intestines, and mid-back.
Essential oils: ginger, Roman chamomile, the Digestive blend, and the Renewing blend.

Low self-worth/lack of self-esteem. Low self-worth or a lack of self-esteem affects vision, the pancreas, the spleen, the midback, and the skin.
Essential oils: bergamot, coriander, lemon, the Anti-aging blend, and the Invigorating blend.

Need to control/out of control. Feeling lack of control affects the bladder, reproductive organs, and sinuses.
Essential oils: basil, cinnamon, cypress, eucalyptus, juniper berry, and the Women's monthly blend.

Resentment. Resentment affects the throat, mouth, and thyroid gland.
Essential oils: clove, lavender, sandalwood, the Protective blend, and the Reassuring blend.

Sadness/grief/depression. Sadness, grief, and prolonged depression affect the heart, lungs, and immune system.
Essential oils: cardamom, eucalyptus, lime, rosemary, ylang ylang, the Comforting blend, and the Respiratory blend.

CHANGING OUR THOUGHTS WITH AFFIRMATIONS

Affirmations are positive assertions, phrased in the present tense, that we repeat to help us reprogram our minds and moods to be more positive and life enhancing. I find the power of essential oils is heightened when combined with affirmations. I suggest you try it yourself and see if you get similar results.

THE FOUR-STEP EMOTIONS MENTORTM METHOD

You have the capacity to take charge of your inner reality using essential oils in combination with affirmations. The quick technique I teach is easy to master.

STEP 1.
Name an emotion you currently have and want to change, or an emotion you want to promote.

Example A: "I want to stop feeling afraid."
Example B: "I want to feel more peaceful."

STEP 2.
Choose an oil that is related to that emotion. Apply it topically or diffuse it.

Example A: Lavender reduces fear. (Refer to "Negative Emotions and Oils That May Support Them" on page 14.)
Example B: Lavender promotes peace. (Refer to "Positive Emotions and Oils That May Promote Them" on page 12.)

STEP 3.

Say an affirmation to change your thoughts or to express the new and better way you want to feel.

Look up the oil you have chosen in the alphabetical guide to oils that begins on page 25. In our example, we selected Lavender. Under the description of this oil, you would find the following affirmations.

Pick one. Say it while you are inhaling your chosen essential oil.

Example: "I freely express my authentic truth."

STEP 4.

Feel your next emotion. Allow yourself to feel your emotions fully and release each of them afterward.

Trust that this energy in motion (e + motion) carries your life force. Be kind and loving no matter what comes up.

WORKING WITH EMOTIONAL POLARITIES

Body, mind, and emotions are linked. So, when you heal a negative state of mind/mood, your body gets healthier.

The medical traditions of many ancient civilizations around the world view the body as a map of connections. In Ayurveda, which comes from India, the grid lines of the physical map are known as *nadis.* In Traditional Chinese Medicine, the gridlines are known as *meridians.*

For our purposes, we should ask: Which organs and physical systems correspond to which emotions?

Lungs/respiratory system = happy/sad
Colon/kidneys/bladder/adrenal glands = calm/fearful
Shoulders/skeletal system = supported/burdened

Brain/nervous system = important/prideful
Liver/gallbladder/circulatory system = strong/angry
Stomach/gut/digestive system = self-worthy/ guilty

On the six-sided Emotions Mentor™ Wheel on the following page, you can find a list of oils and affirmations to promote positive shifts and improve your health overall.

Now, you are empowered to make the most out of your time spent with the individual essential oils and oil blends.

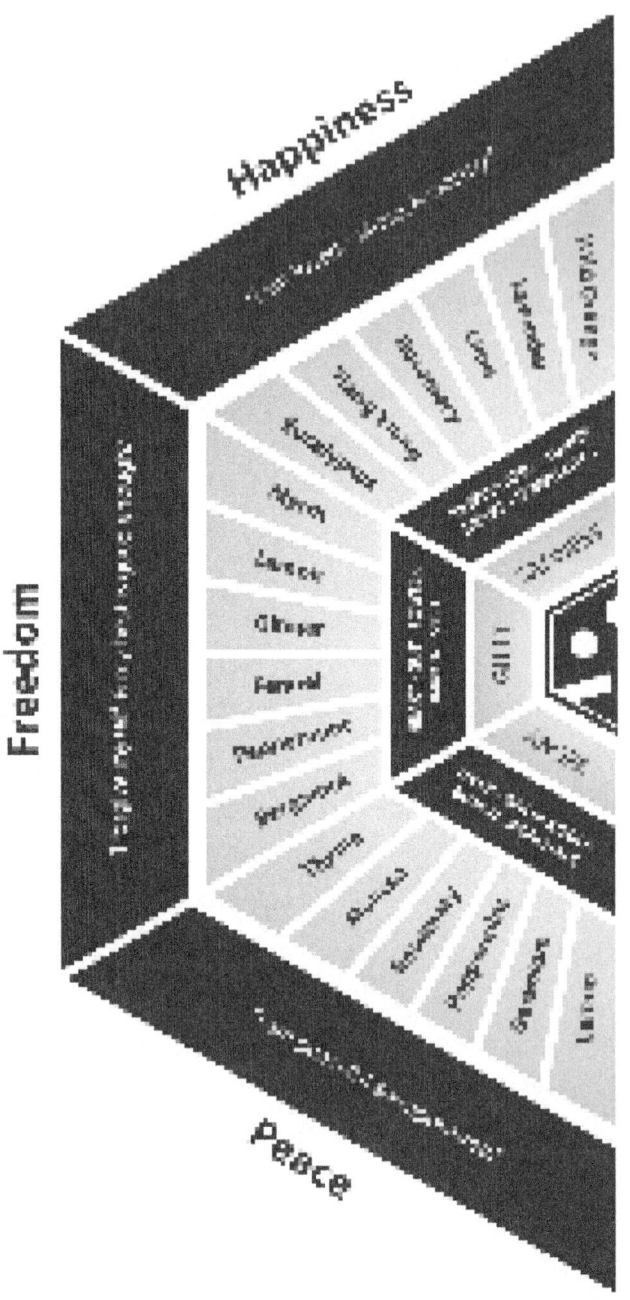

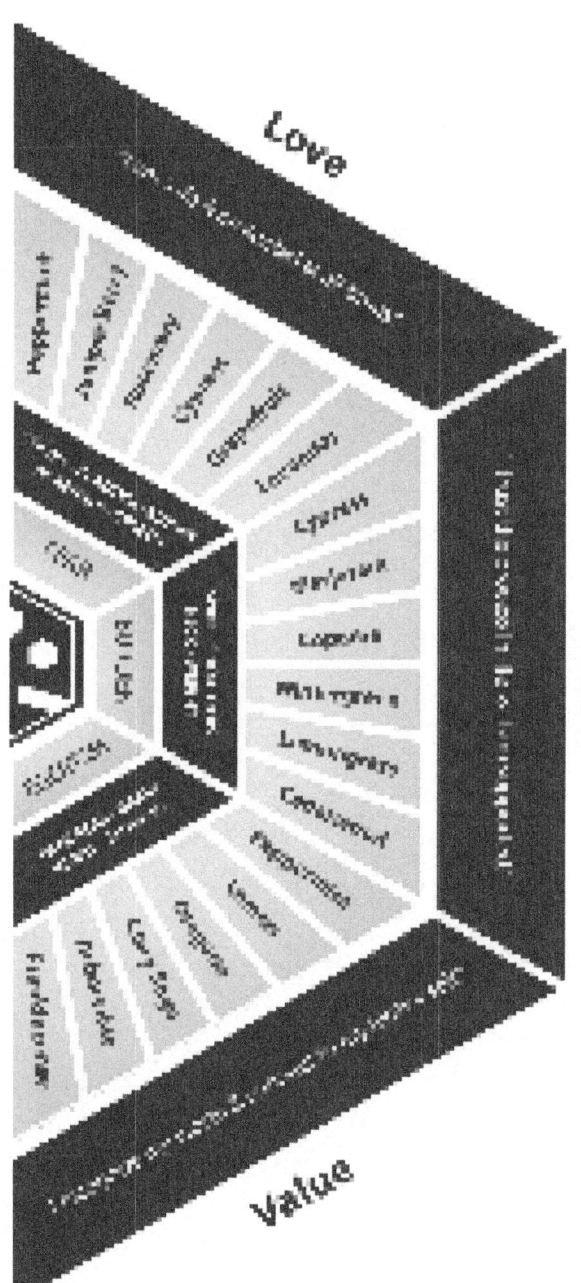

INDIVIDUAL
ESSENTIAL OILS

Accompanying each entry that follows is general information about the oil, emotional states it may benefit, and suggested affirmations. The oils are listed alphabetically by their common names.

Note: Oils may be used aromatically, topically, and/ or internally (only when it is specified that it is safe to do so on the product labels on their packaging). Some require dilution with a carrier oil, such as almond oil, coconut oil, grapeseed oil, or jojoba oil, when they are applied directly on the skin.

A

ARBORVITAE *(Thuja plicata).*

Arborvitae is a member of the tree family. It is grounding and stabilizing to the nervous system. Because it has antiviral, antibacterial, and antifungal properties, it protects and sustains those who use it. Arborvitae is a hearty plant that produces a high yield of essential oil. It may be used to support those who feel broken or ill due to relationships that have been abusive or where there are patterns of codependency. It can be helpful to those facing divorce. If you need additional resources to sustain your strength, better personal boundaries, and a stronger connection to life, arborvitae may provide that added support. It may leave you feeling capable, sturdy, grounded, powerful, and independent.

Emotions: Uncertainty, instability, fear, sadness loneliness, agitation.

Affirmations: I am whole and healthy. I am confident and capable. I accept and love myself as I am. I am able to respond to my needs and the circumstances of my life in healthy and appropriate ways. I am centered and grounded. I am connected to life everywhere.

B

BASIL *(Ocimum basilicum).*

Basil is a member of the mint family. As an herb, it has strong medicinal properties, making it an excellent choice for the treatment of flu and infections. It can also be used to treat mental exhaustion and poor memory. Basil helps renew the mind and restore energy to the body. Its positive properties may help to reprogram the type of emotional patterns that underlie different addictions. Basil can restore hope to the soul.

Emotions: Anger, anxiety, stress, fear.

Affirmations: I am enough. I am peaceful. I release all fears and transform them to faith. I am safe and everything works out for me.

BERGAMOT *(Citrus bergamia).*

A member of the citrus family, bergamot is an excellent choice for uplifting our moods. For those with low self-esteem, bergamot may help restore confidence, hope, and self-assurance. Bergamot supports us to let go of negative thinking and release tension. It also encourages us to connect to who we really are so we may share our authentic selves with others. Applied to the throat, solar plexus, and the bottoms of the feet, bergamot can assist with a good night's sleep. When diffused, it helps create a peaceful environment. Combine bergamot with lime and sandalwood to promote a sense of worthiness and belonging.

Emotions: Self-doubt, discouragement, self-hatred, disappointment, discouragement, stress.

Affirmations: I love and accept myself. I love who I am. I am worthy and important, confident and capable. I am comfortable being me.

BIRCH *(Betula lenta).*

Birch is a member of the tree family. Distilled from bark, its properties are soothing for the soul as well as for pain and inflammation in the body. Birch is helpful for those who feel they are unsupported by the people around them. When we feel alone, birch can comfort us and provide us with strength. It offers sustenance by helping us feel rooted enough to face the storms of life. It also gives us sufficient buoyancy that we may stand alone. Physically, birch provides support to our structural systems—our muscles and bones.

Emotions: Fear, worry, pain, anger, instability, disconnection.

Affirmations: I am supported. I am grounded and stable. I am connected to my life's purpose. I release the past and make room for stable growth. I allow myself to be and feel comforted.

BLACK PEPPER *(Piper nigrum).*

Black pepper is a spice with potent antiviral properties when taken internally, on an emotional level it is helpful in eliminating the "virus" of negative thinking. It pulls up suppressed emotions so they can be dealt with honestly, promoting recovery from addiction and encouraging new ways of thought. Black pepper helps us let go of the old and increases our capacity for the new. It may help those who bottle up emotions to release destructive feelings.

Emotions: Fear, anxiety, overwhelm, self-criticism, doubt.

Affirmations: I am free to choose. It is safe to feel. I am able to peacefully and fearlessly face the truth of my past and my present, and my feelings about it. I accept that I am healing one day at a time.

BLUE TANSY *(Tanacetum annum).*

Boasting a fragrant, mellow, and somewhat fruity scent, blue tansy stands apart from other oils due to its rich and vibrant blue hue. Surprisingly, the plant from which the precious oil is distilled has long, sage-colored stems with hairy leaves and—at the right time of year—tiny clusters of yellow flowers. No blue anywhere! The rich coloring comes from a high concentration of chamazulene that forms when the plant's flowers, leaves, and stems undergo steam distillation. Chamazulene is common in chamomile plants but not at the same high levels it is in blue tansy. Chamazulene is particularly helpful in soothing irritated skin and is high in anti-inflammatory properties. Blue tansy oil is also rich in sabinene, a compound known to reduce blemishes and function as an antioxidant. The oil is potent and effective: just a drop or two mixed with lotion or your favorite carrier oil can be rubbed into sore muscles, smoothed over facial blemishes, or added to a daily cleanser to soothe the skin and awaken the senses in a warm bath or shower. Its aroma is emotionally comforting and mood-lifting.

Emotions: Irritability, stress, anxiety, exhaustion, feeling overworked

Affirmations: I am letting go of worries, fears, and anxiety. Tension in my body and mind melts away as I center myself on those things that matter most.

C

CARDAMOM *(Elettaria cardamomum).*

Made from seeds of a plant in the ginger family, cardamom has a refreshing and invigorating aroma. A versatile spice used in cooking around the world, it stimulates digestion and helps clear channels in the kidneys, making it a tonic for overall health. When we are physically well, our spirits are uplifted and our minds become clearer. Because cardamom stimulates blood flow, it has a warming effect. This effect helps clear congestion from the lungs and may also help overcome conditions such as impotence.

Emotions: Confusion, depression, grief, resistance, frustration.

Affirmations: I am focused and intentional in everything I do. My mind is alert and I am inspired to do great things. My actions are aligned with my best interests. I am able to envision a bright future.

CASSIA *(Cinnamomum cassia).*

Cassia is an oil of courage for those who are shy and hold themselves back. It helps rid us of fear and replace it with self-confidence by helping us recognize our talents and potential. Cassia is also medicinal in nature and can assist in helping those who feel overrun by life to regain inner strength. Cassia is high in cinnamaldehyde, and as such, has been shown to be useful for killing different strains of bacteria, particularly those associated with Lyme disease.

Emotions: Shyness, anxiety, self-doubt, timidity, overwhelm.

Affirmations: I courageously face my destiny. I enthusiastically share my gifts and talents with the world. I am safe to let others see and know the real me. My strength is building day by day.

CEDARWOOD *(Juniperus virginiana).*
Cedarwood helps those who struggle to form social connections. It opens the heart so we may feel the love and support of others. It helps us to feel like we belong and rid our souls of impressions of loneliness and isolation. Cedarwood belongs to the conifer tree family, and as such, it's soothing to the central nervous system. Consequently, cedarwood can be used topically on the bottoms of feet along with lavender and/or Roman chamomile to support a good night's sleep. It is also purifying and sedative.

Emotions: Depression, anxiety, irritability, confusion, loneliness.

Affirmations: I am calm and secure. I am safe to connect. My heart opens to receive love. I am deeply supported. Life is on my side.

CILANTRO *(Coriandrum sativum).*
Cilantro is a type of parsley. It comes from the same plant as coriander, but is extracted differeently—by steam distillation from the leaves. High in antioxidants that protect our cells from oxidative stress, it also helps us cleanse ourselves of the negative emotions that weigh down the body. It's a natural detoxifier, physically and emotionally. It can help us interrupt patterns of rigid, destructive behavior and lighten our emotional load, allowing us to return to our true selves.

Cilantro may be supportive for migraine headaches and riding the body of heavy metal toxicity.

Emotions: *Rigidity, resistance, self-hatred, irritability, anger, stress.*

Affirmations: *I am in flow. I am effortlessly releasing thoughts and feelings that do not serve me. My mind and heart are untouched by negativity around me. Positive energy uplifts me unceasingly.*

CHAMOMILE. ROMAN. *(See Roman chamomile)*

CINNAMON *(Cinnamomum zeylanicum).*
Distilled from bark, cinnamon essential oil is a spice oil that is helpful in regulating blood sugar. It has antibacterial and immune-boosting properties. It promotes well-being by supporting healthy digestion. Emotionally, it restores joy and supports sexual health. It encourages us to be honest and vulnerable in our relationships, allowing intimacy to flourish, while also supporting us in sustaining healthy boundaries. It also has been known to rekindle desire that has been lost due to trauma or abuse.

Emotions: *Depression, mental exhaustion, post-trauma, low libido.*

Affirmations: *My mind is sharp and my body is healthy. I am able to set and sustain healthy personal boundaries with the people in my life. I am able to trust myself. I allow myself to experience intimacy.*

CLARY SAGE *(Salvia sclaria).*

Clary sage is a member of the mint family. It promotes clarity of mind and helps us to open our psyches to new ideas and perspectives. It supports creativity by increasing our ability to focus and visualize. It can also help us better develop our spiritual gifts. Physically, it interacts with the body's hormonal system, and can, therefore, bring hormonal balance and stimulate interest in intimacy. Women entering menopause may find it useful to combine clary sage with geranium (topically) to support mood and hormonal balance.

Emotions: Mood swings, disconnection, depression, low libido, stress.

Affirmations: I trust myself completely. I remain calm, cool, and collected at all times. I am a powerful creator. I am focused and persistent. My mind and my heart are aligned with my intentions.

CLOVE *(Eugenia caryophyllata).* Clove is a powerful antioxidant that has many medicinal uses, including the treatment of toothaches, digestive upsets, parasites, and arthritis. Emotionally, clove supports us in establishing healthy boundaries in relationships. It gives individuals with a tendency to feel victimized and out of control a sense of personal power. It supports us in being able to do what is necessary to protect ourselves.

Emotions: Fear, helplessness, overwhelm, anxiety, selfdoubt.

Affirmations: I am confident and capable. I am in charge of my destiny. I believe in myself and my abilities. Everything works out well for me.

COPAIBA *(Copaifera).*

Steam extracted from the resinous balsam that flows naturally from trees of the same name, copaiba has been used medicinally for centuries. As early as the 1500s, natives of Northern and Northeastern Brazil began harvesting the oil from 100-foot tall copaiba trees deep in the Amazon. Then and now, the spicy, woodsy oil has been used to treat a wide variety of symptoms concerning nearly all of the major body systems. The main chemical component of copaiba—caryophyllene—works with cell receptors in the body to provide effective pain relief, support the digestive, cardiovascular, immune, and nervous systems, and even act as an antibacterial agent. Copaiba oil can soothe both irritated skin and troubled minds. Emotionally, copaiba assists us in uncovering negative emotions and unhealthy patterns that we've carried for many years, perhaps even for generations, in our families. Just as it helps physical digestion, it can also help us improve the way we digest and process life as it supports a peace of mind that wipes away the roots of what trouble our souls and helps us move forward with confidence.

Emotions: Fear, regret, shame, anger, distrust.

Affirmations: I am capable and strong. I can clear my mind of shame and fear and move forward with my life. The past does not determine who I am today.

CORIANDER *(Coriandrum sativum).*

Coriander oil comes from the same plant as cilantro, but is distilled from the seeds. Coriander is an excellent support for those of us who are people-pleasers or who have lost sight of who we are and can't find joy in the lives we've created. It is also especially useful for emotional eaters. Emotionally, it teaches us that we can be happy as we are and do not need to repress our emotions. Often, we grow up believing we must please others to be loved, and thus, happy. When there is no joy in life, at times, we may turn to sugar and sweets to make us feel better. Coriander supports us in being loyal to ourselves by encouraging us to do the things that are in alignment with the true self. Physically, coriander is helpful for blood sugar imbalances. A therapeuticgrade drop of coriander may be taken internally to support the body when there's been too much sugar intake. It's also useful to rub coriander directly over the pancreas.

Emotions: *Sadness, flatness, instability, anxiety, suppression, anger.*

Affirmations: *I allow myself to feel my feelings. I love and accept myself. I affirm my right to stand my ground when people disagree with me. My needs are always taken care of effortlessly.*

CYPRESS *(Cupressus sempervirens).*

Cypress oil supports the free flow of energy. Individuals who feel emotionally stuck may find cypress a great resource. It encourages us to be more flexible and let go of control. It's also tremendously helpful for bringing up and then releasing deeply stored pain. As a member of the tree family, it provides emotional grounding. Physically, cypress is supportive to the circulatory system—improving the flow of blood and lymph. It strengthens the structural systems of the body: bones, muscles, and soft tissues.

Emotions: *Loss, fear, resistance, uneasiness, trauma, depression.*

Affirmations: *I am flexible and free. I am grounded and centered. The energy of the universe flows through me and promotes the good of all. Obstacles in my path and around me are dissolving effortlessly.*

D

DILL *(Anethum graveolens).*

An herb in the parsley family, dill promotes purification of the body, digestion, and healthy nervous system functioning. When we're in a heightened emotional state or being challenged, it can help us stay calm. In situations where we feel we are being unfairly treated or we are having a hard time accepting reality, dill oil can help us to "digest" or process our emotions successfully.

Emotions: Stress, anxiety, depression, agitation, overexcitement.

Affirmations: I accept what is without feeling diminished in any way by it. I remain peaceful and relaxed always. I feel happy to be alive.

DOUGLAS FIR *(Pseudotsuga menziesii).*

A highly fragrant tree oil used medicinally by Native Americans and long associated with the celebration of Christmas, Douglas fir promotes mental clarity and creativity, and elevates our moods. It naturally revitalizes the spirits and soothes the soul. Douglas fir oil promotes healthy respiration and can also reduce muscular pain and stiffness—thereby making us feel good. When we use it, we experience a sense of general well-being. Those who tend to become scattered in their thinking or are easily distractible, due to ADHD or chaotic circumstances, find it restores their focus.

Emotions: Depression, futility, loss, stress, mental fatigue.

Affirmations: My mind is alert and I am focused on my goals. I easily accomplish anything I set my mind on doing. My spirit is uplifted and I am filled with the energy for living. I love expressing my creativity.

E

EUCALYPTUS *(Eucalyptus radiata).*

Eucalyptus has been used for centuries to support the respiratory system. In promoting easy breathing, eucalyptus supports healing and wellness. In particular, eucalyptus seems to tap into the emotions of those who have a pattern of illness and helps them move forward to living in wellness. It encourages us all to face our issues head on and let go of negative emotions. Eucalyptus is grounding and soothing to the soul and silently suggests a renewal of life and good health to an ailing body and spirit.

Emotions: Anger, oversensitivity, grief, resistance, stress, frustration.

Affirmations. As I breathe, I sense all the obstructions in my life dissolving effortlessly. My soul is soothed as I remember to breathe. I am connected to the life force that animates everything in the universe.

F

FENNEL *(Foeniculum vulgare).*

Historically, fennel has been used to promote digestive wellness. It's also known to support hormonal balance. And just as fennel supports digestion, it helps us digest the process of life. It strengthens our souls to imagine that the desires of the heart can be obtained. Fennel supports us when we feel overwhelmed by reminding us of our potential, helping us reconnect with our inner selves, and inspiring remembrance of a bigger perspective.

Emotions: Stress, depression, overwhelm, frustration, fear.

Affirmations: I boldly step forward into my future. Everything I desire is mine. My potential is unlimited.

FIR. DOUGLAS. *(See Douglas fir)*

FRANKINCENSE *(Boswellia frereana, B. carteri, B. sacra).*

Frankincense is often referred to as the "father" of all essential oils because it has so many applications. This oil helps us to connect to our inner spirits. It helps rid us of spiritual darkness and mental deception by helping us see the light within and remember our talents and potential. It improves our attitudes and intuition. Also, frankincense reminds us that we are loved and not forgotten. Frankincense is helpful for anyone who is struggling with issues with a father, either temporal or spiritual.

Emotions: *Fear, shame, disappointment, insecurity, selfdoubt.*

Affirmations: *I trust myself and I remain calm at all times. I am safe. I am supported and unconditionally loved. My needs are being met.*

G

GERANIUM *(Pelargonium graveolens).*
Geranium soothes a broken heart and powerfully releases past baggage. It helps individuals who have lost hope in people and the world around them. Geranium reminds the soul that the world is mostly good and most people have good intentions. It also brings up the pain of the past so one can work through old emotions and begin to see all that's good. Geranium may be combined with clary sage to bring hormonal balance (and thus mood balance) to women during menopause. Combine with lime oil if you are working to release deeply rooted emotional wounds.

Emotions: *Loss, disappointment, fear, depression, mistrust.*

Affirmations: *I am kind and patient with myself and others. The world is a safe place. I am patient with my healing process. Every experience gives me an opportunity to love myself and others more.*

GINGER *(Zingiber officinale).*

Ginger is the ultimate encourager. It helps us to live in the present and seize the day. It empowers us to achieve the potential we were destined to fulfill. Just as ginger oil promotes physical digestion, it encourages healthy digestion of uncomfortable challenges and supports resolution of gut-related anxiety.

Emotions: Anxiety, stress, fear, obstinacy, doubt, complacency.

Affirmations: I am fired about my plans and ready to meet my challenges head on. I am present and alert. I love to express myself creatively. I am a powerful creator with an important destiny to fulfill. I digest the process of life. I am nurtured and supported.

GRAPEFRUIT *(Citrus x paradisi).*

Grapefruit is a member of the citrus family, and as such, a natural mood uplifter. Historically, grapefruit oil has been used topically (diluted) to reduce fat from problem areas of the body because it cleanses toxins from fatty cells. Consequently, it is a great essential oil for individuals who are unhappy because they can't seem ever to be satisfied with the way they look. Grapefruit helps us love our bodies more by inspiring us to pay attention to what our bodies really need. It also may help control appetite. Because it can improve hormonal balance, it helps to eliminate "toxic" thoughts relating to self-worth. When combined with cassia and inhaled, grapefruit can increase our confidence in ourselves and our appearance.

Emotions: Self-hatred, dissatisfaction, negativity, depression, anxiety.

GREEN MANDARIN *(Citrus nobilis).*

Green mandarin essential oil is unique in that the oil is cold pressed from the unripe and typically discarded fruit of the mandarin tree. To effectively grow mandarin trees that produce a healthy, vibrant crop, the trees must be heavily thinned while the fruit is still young and green. This means that much of the young fruit is plucked from the tree and never goes on to ripen and be counted as part of a successful mandarin crop. Rather than having the green fruit go to waste, farmers in Brazil have found that its peel can be cold pressed to produce a wonderful, fragrant oil with cleansing, emotionally stabilizing, and purifying properties. With its sweet, refreshing scent, green mandarin oil can uplift emotions and relieve negative energy from around or within you. Like other oils in the citrus family, it can help relieve symptoms of depression. Diffusing it in the home helps to purify the air and eliminate unpleasant odors. Adding a few drops to your facial toner and swiping it across your face can tone and clarify skin. And because the oil comes from fruit that is young and unripe and has therefore not yet developed measurable levels of furanocoumarins, it does not carry a photosensitivity warning like other citrus oils do.

Emotions: Negativity, depression, melancholy, bitterness, rejection.

Affirmations: I welcome positivity into my life. I am patient and kind to myself. I am learning to let go of the negative and embrace the good. Each day is a fresh start.

H

HAWAIIAN SANDALWOOD
(Santalum paniculatum).
Hawaiian sandalwood is very calming and stabilizing. It harmonizes our emotions and gives us mental clarity and the intuition. Many people find that Hawaiian sandalwood enhances meditation.

Emotions: Stress, anxiety, low libido, depression, lack of focus.

Affirmations: I am beautiful inside and out. It is comfortable for me to openly reveal my authentic self and express my truth. With every breath and every step, I increase my peace. All is well.

HELICHRYSUM *(Helichrysum italicum).*
Helichrysum is the ultimate essential oil for healing deep emotional pain, which it helps by addressing the emotions that are behind the pain. Helichrysum helps restore the love for living that individuals who have been weighed down by agony feel, because it encourages the restoration of belief. It is useful for those struggling with addiction when they experience self-rejection and self-hatred. It may be useful to rub helichrysum over the liver, as the liver is the organ that is traditionally associated with painful emotions like anger, fear, and hate.

Emotions: Anger, fear, hatred, depression, selfrecrimination.

J

JASMINE *(Jasminum officinale).*

Jasmine is a fragrant essential oil with a sweet scent that has long been associated with romance because the jasmine flower blooms only at night. Jasmine oil is pleasing and emotionally elevating, and may stimulate the release of serotonin and other hormones, resulting in a surge of energy and a sense of overall wellbeing. Jasmine opens the heart and paves the way for improved intimacy for couples who have grown distant, and it makes it easier for those who are drawn together out of attraction to trust one another. Jasmine oil is calming and may help promote undisturbed sleep. It is also good for the skin and for relieving self-consciousness.

Emotions: Anxiety, disconnection, self-consciousness, mistrust, stress.

Affirmations: I am safe to love freely. I trust myself. I am open to new experiences. Sleep is my friend.

JUNIPER BERRY *(Juniperus communis).*

Juniper berry is an excellent resource for the bladder and kidneys. It's often used to treat kidney and urinary tract infections. Emotionally, juniper berry helps those who are ridden by fear, anger, and a lack of security in life. Juniper berry suggests to the mind and body ways to work through the underlying issues that create intense fear and anger. It helps one feel protected and have the courage to face life with the knowledge that it's possible to create peace, balance, and a sense of security.

Emotions: Fear, anger, distrust, stress, grief, holding back.

Affirmations: I release that which no longer serves me. I am willing to forgive myself and others for being human. I accept that I am doing the best I can. I feel peaceful and protected. All is well.

L

LAVENDER *(Lavandula angustifolia).*
Lavender is the oil of communication. It enhances cellular communication and also encourages honest communication. It helps individuals express their true selves. Lavender is a powerful anti-inflammatory. It is calming and soothing to the central nervous system and can dramatically help reduce symptoms of anxiety. It is sometimes considered the mother of all essential oils, offering some of the broadest medicinal uses, from treating burns and bug bites, to reducing joint pain and helping eliminate headaches.

Emotions: Stress, agitation, anger, fear, anxiety, distrust.

Affirmations: I freely express my authentic truth. Opportunities are everywhere for me when I am ready. I am relaxed and at ease in every situation. I am at peace with my body. I accept and love myself as I am.

LEMON *(Citrus limon).*

Lemon is a natural mood uplifter. Its clean, fresh scent lightens the environment and encourages cleanliness and emotional housekeeping. Lemon supports individuals who have learning disabilities or find it hard to focus. It assists us in finding clarity and choosing to live in the present moment, focusing on one thing at a time. It also restores confidence in those who have negative self-thoughts associated with learning. Lemon is also highly antibacterial and can be used as a natural hand sanitizer while uplifting mood immediately when inhaled.

Emotions: *Self-doubt, anxiety, confusion, frustration, overwhelm.*

Affirmations: I am capable of greatness. I am able and willing to learn. I love myself unconditionally. It is a joy to contribute my gifts and talents to the world. My future is bright. I am perfectly supported and nurtured to grow into my full potential.

LEMON BALM. *(See Melissa)*

LEMONGRASS *(Cymbopogon flexuosus).*

Lemongrass is a fantastic emotional house cleaner (assuming the body is the house of our emotions). It supports individuals who feel stagnant in life to clear the clutter and move forward. It helps energy to flow freely so we can live with confidence. Lemongrass can bridge the gap between desires of the heart and mind. Physically, it is helpful for bringing balance to the thyroid system. It's highly antimicrobial, anti-infectious, and helpful at increasing circulation, so it's often taken internally to promote wellness.

Emotions: Fear, negativity, self-criticism, doubt, lack of drive.

Affirmations: When my intentions are clear, the universe cooperates with me and I can accomplish anything. I am always successful. Success is in my blood. Life is beautiful. Life is fulfilling. I love life.

LIME *(Citrus aurantifolia).*

Lime, a member of the citrus family, lifts mood, supports the respiratory system, and helps individuals feel joy by helping rid negative emotions like depression and discouragement. It instills love and happiness back into the heart. It's wonderful for releasing grief and pain. Combined with geranium, lime can wipe away the barnacles and clear the path, making way for beneficial changes.

Emotions: Anxiety, anger, depression, discouraged, mental fatigue.

Affirmations: I feel energized and uplifted by my life. Joy is my name and gratitude is the nature of my game. I am easily releasing negativity.

LITSEA *(Litsea cubeba).*

Citrusy, sweet, and spicy all at once, litsea essential oil is produced by steam distilling the tiny pepper-like buds of the litsea cubeba, commonly known as a may chang tree. May chang, an evergreen native to Southeast Asia and often called Mountain Pepper, is from the laurel family, and its buds are considered a spice despite their citrus-like fragrance. The oil is used for everything from manufacturing soaps and perfumes to promoting the health of the cardiovascular, immune, nervous, and respiratory systems. Litsea oil can be diffused or inhaled to calm nerves and tackle anxiety.

When topically applied, it is both cleansing and healing. Massaging the oil over the stomach can reduce digestive symptoms such as cramping and flatulence. Mixing a few drops with moisturizer or lotion and smoothing over the face can clear blemishes and clean clogged pores. Inhaling it can be energizing and refreshing.

Emotions: *Stress, frustration, a cloudy mind, discomfort.*

Affirmations: *I am mentally present. My mind is clear and I am able to think through problems and overcome setbacks. I have control over my thoughts.*

M

MAGNOLIA *(Michelia x alba).*
More than 200 varieties of magnolia are present on the earth, most found in Asia and the Americas. These flowering trees are said to have existed even before bees did, being pollinated instead by beetles. Because of the tree's endurance, its blooms are considered sacred by many ancient cultures and are often used in ceremonial events, such as weddings. The blooms tend to be sturdier than most flowers and can be harvested several times throughout a year. Magnolia oil is distilled from blossoms that are handpicked early in the morning or late in the evening when their petals' fragrance is at its height and they are ideal for extracting the compelling, floral oil. Because it is high in linalool, magnolia essential

oil carries a pleasant, soothing, and relaxing scent. When diluted with a carrier oil and applied to the wrists or the back of the neck, the oil assists wearers in expressing feelings of compassion, forgiveness, and communication while decreasing irritability and envy.

Emotions: *Irritability, envy, jealousy, frustration, anger, sleeplessness.*

Affirmations: *I am proud of my own accomplishments and do not need to compare myself to others. Happiness does not come from being better than others or having more. Happiness comes when I am being my best self.*

MANUKA *(Leptospermum scoparium).*

Steam distilled from the leaves and branches of the prolific flowering manuka tree in New Zealand, manuka essential oil has been used for centuries to heal and soothe. Natives have traditionally used all parts of the manuka tree for a wide variety of purposes. Leaves are steamed and the vapors inhaled to treat colds and congestion; sawdust from manuka wood is used to add flavor to meats and fish when smoked; a mixture of its bark and leaves is made to rub over stiff, sore muscles; honey is produced by bees who feast on nectar from manuka's flowers; the tree's bark is chewed to promote sleep; essential oil from the tree is antibacterial, cleansing, and soothing and can be used to treat dandruff, athlete's foot, and skin irritations. No part of this precious plant goes to waste! Manuka essential oil has properties similar to those in melaleuca, or tea tree, oil. In fact, the manuka is often called the New Zealand tea tree, and both trees are part of the myrtle family. Manuka trees grow quickly and will regenerate swiftly as natural clearing of the land takes place. As such, the oil from the tree is said to support change, growth, and the birth of new ideas.

Emotions: Fear, instability, discomfort, ambivalence.

Affirmations: I welcome change and growth each day. I look forward to new experiences, new relationships, and new opportunities to grow.

MARJORAM *(Origanum majorana).*

Marjoram relieves joint and tissue pain, particularly when combined with lemongrass. Alone, marjoram helps individuals who cannot create meaningful relationships, because of deep emotional wounds or trauma, to move forward and connect. Marjoram can assist in helping us learn to trust others and ourselves. It is a member of the mint family, and as such, it has antibacterial and antiviral properties making it medicinal in nature.

Emotions: Anger, depression, self-doubt, fear, loneliness.

Affirmations: I am a good person. I am strong, courageous, and brave. I am not alone today. The trauma/ abuse/ betrayal was not my fault. I trust myself. My life has a beautiful meaning and a higher purpose.

MELISSA *(Melissa officinalis).*

Melissa is also known as lemon balm. Melissa is a powerful support to the human brain. It is also highly antiviral, and thus supports freeing the body of unwanted programming that affects healthy thinking. Melissa is sometimes referred to as the oil of truth. It helps individuals see who they really are and why they are here. It can support spiritual connection. It encourages one to press on through the hard times and love their life. It is a strong supporter of relieving depressive symptoms and recovering from traumas that have impacted the brain.

Emotions: Disconnection, depression, trauma, anger, negativity.

Affirmations: Obstacles are now falling away easily. I have a right to my feelings. Today, I welcome health and happiness. I abandon old habits and choose new, positive ones. I am the authority on my own experience. I deserve love, success, and fulfillment in great measure.

MYRRH *(Commiphora myrrha).*

Myrrh essential oil is made from the distilled resin and gum of a tree. It is an extraordinary preservative that was used by ancient Egyptians for embalming, and as such, is excellent for the skin. Myrrh oil balances the thyroid system, which regulates our metabolic processes; it also helps heal subconscious conflicts and encourages nurturing self-expression. It also supports healthy gums and mouth care. Just as myrrh can be used at birth to help heal the cutting of an umbilical cord of a newborn, it can help heal relationships, specifically a hardened relationship between a mother and her child. Myrrh helps the child within each of us feel safe and loved, filling any void in our mother/child relationship. Myrrh supports meditation.

Emotions: Anger, shame, disconnection, depression.

Affirmations: I am in perfect communion with the wholeness of creation. I am completely true to myself, alive and empowered, fully and freely creative. I am sheltered by the mercy of spirit/God/the universe. I am divinely led and guided in all I think, do, and say.

N

NEROLI *(Citrus aurantium).*

The exotic, sweet, and florally tones of neroli oil come from steam distilling the small white flowers of the bitter orange tree. The flowers are handpicked at peak bloom and processed right away to prevent the petals from being bruised or handled too heavily. The bitter orange tree also yields bitter orange oil, which is extracted from the fruit's peel, and petitgrain, which is extracted from the tree's leaves. Neroli, because of its labor-intensive extraction, is considered the most precious of the three oils—and the rarest of the citrus oils. Its pleasing, bright, and florally aroma has the power to drastically uplift the mood and soothe the mind. When applied topically, it is also soothes the skin and helps revive dull and dry tones. If needed, neroli can be diffused in a room to spark creativity and make life feel less dull. Neroli eases feelings of anxiety, stress, and even depression. It comforts and relaxes the body and mind to promote overall wellness. Applying topically or diffusing throughout the day will diminish negative or overwhelming thoughts swirling in your head. Pairing the oil with lavender can boost these effects.

Emotions: Stress, anxiety, discouragement, dullness

Affirmations: Divine inspiration flows through me. I am well, whole, creative, and capable. My mind is free and open.

O

ORANGE. WILD. *(See Wild orange)*

OREGANO *(Origanum vulgare).*

Oregano is a very powerful essential oil that can relieve pain and infection. It can get through to individuals who are stubborn and hold tightly to unhealthy belief systems. Its strong medicinal properties work similarly to prescription antibiotics. Metaphorically, oregano works similarly on our emotional system, fighting convincingly for the body's sound emotional health by eliminating unwanted thoughts and patterns. Oregano makes a strong statement to let go of toxic attachments, bad relationships, and sabotaging habits, thus making it easier to move forward in life.

Emotions: Obsession, resistance, negativity, competition, jealousy.

Affirmations: The more I focus my mind on the good, the more good comes to me. I trust I am being led to where I need to be. My life is important. I can change the world just by being here, right now. I surrender my ego and no longer let fear and envy rule my life.

P

PATCHOULI *(Pogostemon cablin).*

Patchouli is a grounding essential oil that helps stabilize the central nervous system. It fosters communication between the heart and body so that they can work better together. It also supports us in letting go of negative thoughts about life and reminds us to find beauty in the world around us. Patchouli can cross the blood-brain barrier to chemically support the brain and nervous system. Patchouli can aid in addiction recovery, as it works to shift our mindset and reestablish a healthy connection to life.

Emotions: Anxiety, regret, self-doubt, worry, depression, insecurity.

Affirmations: I am surrounded by people who love and support me, and I love and support myself. I respect myself and know that my opinion and voice matter. I communicate my feelings and needs in healthy, respectful ways. My needs are met easily and effortlessly.

PEPPERMINT *(Mentha piperita).*

Peppermint stimulates the brain and increases circulation. To rapidly increase mood and brain function, combine peppermint with wild orange and inhale. As you do so, you'll find you've increased neuronal activity in your brain (you'll also open your sinuses and breathe more easily), and suddenly you'll feel a wave of happy emotions encompass you. Emotionally, peppermint helps individuals who are struggling with depression to see the joy in life. Peppermint helps to lift sadness and pressure and can put a cap on an overflow of unhealthy emotions. However, we should not use peppermint as a permanent escape. It should be used to help see the joy of life and encourage us to work through the issues holding us back. Peppermint is also good for headaches, memory, and focusing.

Emotions: *Sluggishness, depression, stress, lack of focus, resistance.*

Affirmations: *I am open and receptive to all the abundance life offers me. I can handle massive success with grace. The positive advantage is always mine. My attitude grows happier and healthier every single day.*

PETITGRAIN *(Citrus aurantium).*
Made from the leaves of bitter orange, petitgrain essential oil is an extraordinarily potent mood elevator. It may help stimulate the mind, promote the recall of positive memories, reduce mental fatigue, and ease depression. The scent is vibrant and refreshing. When we use petitgrain, it is like pressing the reset button on a computer screen and opening a new "window" for life to surprise us. As an antioxidant, anti-inflammatory, antibacterial, and anti-infectious compound, petitgrain boosts our immunity. As we heal physically, our moods may stabilize and we may experience more joy being alive.

Emotions: *Depression, irritability, lack of focus, confusion, fatigue.*

Affirmations: *My personality is radiant with confidence, certainty, and optimism. I am always in the right place at the right time. Today is rich with opportunities and I open my heart to receive them. I am joyful.*

PINK PEPPER *(Schinus molle).*

Native to the Peruvian Andes, the Schinus molle is a quick-growing evergreen known for its bright pink berries, which are often called pink peppercorns due to their close resemblance to commercial peppercorn (Piper nigrum). And though the two berries resemble each other—and both carry a peppery scent and flavor—they come from different species of trees. Pink pepper trees are actually more closely related to cashew trees! Ancient Incans used all parts of the tree for healing, religious ceremonies, and culinary use. Today, pink pepper essential oil is known for its ability to support digestive health and maintain a healthy metabolism. A drop added daily to chai tea or water can support the respiratory and immune systems. Some research has indicated that the combination of limonene and a-phellandrene in pink pepper oil can also soothe the nervous system when a drop or two of the oil is diluted in at least four ounces of water and drunk daily. Diffusing pink pepper with a citrus oil brings on feelings of relief and awakens the mind. The oil works on an emotional level to diminish self-doubt and criticism, bring understanding to past problems, and open doors to a new outlook on troubling situations.

Emotions: Self-doubt, exhaustion, fear of change, apprehension, stagnation.

Affirmations: The future is an open book, and I am unafraid to turn its pages. I am strong, worthy, and loved.

R

ROMAN CHAMOMILE *(Anthemis nobilis).*

Roman chamomile helps us feel calm and restores our sense of purpose in life. It is very calming to our minds and bodies, and helps heal broken hearts. Roman chamomile also helps individuals who have lost their sense of who they are to regain their purpose in life. It gives us confidence and the motivation to succeed. Roman chamomile also promotes healthy digestion. For this reason, we know that it can help us digest the emotions we feel.

Emotions: Grief, depression, purposelessness, fear, agitation, shock.

Affirmations: In my sadness, I love myself. All things are unfolding as they are supposed to. I let go of my sorrow, but hold on to my love for my loved ones. I am discovering new strengths within myself.

ROSE *(Rosa damascena).*

Rose encourages spiritual healing by helping us feel divine love. When an individual can connect to divine love, emotional wounds tend to resolve. Rose helps us to connect to love by encouraging connection, prayer, and meditation. When we connect in this way, we often feel more compassion and charity. Rose restores clarity and reestablishes the power of a loving spirit to heal through love. Rose can be useful at both birth and death encounters, bringing great peace and comfort to these substantial transitions in life.

Emotions: Disconnection, depression, fear, envy, grief, shame.

Affirmations: I live skillfully and effectively, and I am steadily awakening to self-realization. I constantly experience and express complete well-being in all aspects of my life. I am invincibly protected against any imperfect suggestion. I am the living embodiment of a divine spirit.

ROSEMARY *(Rosmarinus officinalis).*

Rosemary encourages us to gain greater knowledge by searching for deeper answers. It helps to expand the mind beyond first assumptions. It also helps us feel comfort and confidence in times of change. Rosemary is helpful for adrenal fatigue and mental exhaustion. It helps the respiratory system, and thus aids in lifting the burdens weighing heavily on us. It promotes detoxification.

Emotions: Stress, anxiety, fear, depression, overwhelm, fatigue, grief.

Affirmations: The healing energy of the universe surrounds me and I am restored to perfect health. I am living my life according to my highest vision, which is inspired by love and joy. I am the architect of my life; I build its foundation and choose its contents. I am a radiant being.

S

SANDALWOOD *(Santalum album)*.

Sandalwood assists us in opening our souls to honest and healthy connection. In doing so, it offers clarity and spiritual strengthening. Sandalwood helps to calm the heart and prepares us to talk to God/our higher power. It also allows us to see life in a bigger perspective. It can help us better align our lives with divine purpose. Research on sandalwood suggests that it has powerful properties that aid in restoring healthy cellular function.

Emotions: Confusion, regret, purposelessness, depression, stress.

Affirmations: My nature is divine. I am a spiritual being. Everything that is happening now is happening for my ultimate good. I love myself and I accept myself as I am. I am naturally feminine, graceful and beautiful. I am a woman of love. My touch heals all wounds.

SANDALWOOD. HAWAIIAN.
(See Hawaiian sandalwood).

SIBERIAN FIR *(Abies sibirica)*.

Native to the frigid hills and plains of Siberia, which stretch across Eurasia and North Asia, Siberian fir trees are hardy, strong, and vibrant, able to live more than 100 years in harsh conditions. The oil that is steam extracted from the tree's fragrant needles and twigs promotes similar feelings of strength and vibrancy. Rich in camphene, Siberian fir oil provides respiratory support and facilitates easier, clearer breathing. Deeply inhaling the oil for even a few moments can clear congestion in both the chest and mind. The bornyl acetate in Siberian fir oil is ideal for skin care, and regular use can effectively lighten skin pigmentation. The oil's concentrated amount of alpha-pinene makes it a valuable tool in fighting anxiety and stress. Siberian fir supports emotional stability, harmony of thoughts and feelings, and clarity of mind. It's vibrant, piney smell pairs well with most citrus oils to create a blend that can promote a positive and happy mood.

Emotions: *Confusion, instability, anxiety, stress, exhaustion.*

Affirmations: *I hold on to emotions that elevate and let go of those that denigrate. I am calm and relaxed. My mind is clear and my spirit is grounded in truth.*

SPEARMINT *(Mentha spicata).*

A member of the mint family, the menthol fragrance and taste of spearmint is refreshingly buoyant and rejuvenating. It may bring relief from depression and stagnation of energy.

Emotions: *Stress, anxiety, agitation, over excitement, isolation.*

Affirmations: *The whole process of living makes me happy. I am grateful to God for this wonderful life. I am thankful for everyone who has touched my life and made it worth living. I am kind, I am loving, I am happy.*

SPIKENARD *(Nardostachys jatamansi).*

Spikenard essential oil has been highly prized for thousands of years in the Middle East and the Far East for its far-ranging uses. Complex in composition, it is valued for its ability to foster regeneration of the skin. Emotionally, it assists us when we're in transition between different roles and identities, and undergoing rapid growth as people. Spikenard promotes higher consciousness and opens the third eye so that our powers of intuition may intensify.

Emotions: Disorientation, anxiety, fear, resistance, lack of clarity.

Affirmations: Today I am blessed with absolute clarity. I am on purpose and achieving results. Wisdom guides my vision. I am an expert at keeping my thoughts in order. I feel confident and capable when surfing the waves of change.

T

TANGERINE *(Citrus reticulata).*

Tangerine essential oil is perfect for those who feel burdened by responsibilities that aren't theirs. From the citrus family, tangerine frees us so we can let go and be happy, to find the joy in life and escape debilitating pressures for a period. It also helps to replenish our creative juices. Tangerine is a natural mood uplifter.

Emotions: Overwhelmed, fatigued, depressed, burdened.

Affirmations: My heart leaps with joy the moment my eyes open in the morning. I maintain a continuous attitude of gratitude. Joy is mine right here right now. I choose to be joyful, loving, and inspired.

TEA TREE *(Melaleuca alternifolia).*

Tea Tree oil supports healthy boundaries. It's used medicinally to support daily wellness, reduce unwanted and destructive bacteria, and keep the body fresh and well. For those who have been chronically ill, tea tree rebuilds confidence in life and in good health. It supports us in creating strong boundaries and helps us rid ourselves of negative thoughts of others and ourselves. Tea tree oil can help us desire to stick up for what we believe in and desire.

Emotions: Anger, shame, fear, confusion, resignation.

Affirmations: I can see others' choices as learning experiences without judging. I allow others to experience their own lessons. I am a go-getter and will stop at nothing to achieve my goals. My body is my ally in living the wonderful life of my dreams.

THYME *(Thymus vulgaris).*

Thyme helps release emotions that may be buried deep down, including anger that's been stored for a long time. Bringing unhealthy emotions to the surface helps us process through them and ultimately get rid of them. By ridding our hearts, minds, and bodies of strongly rooted negative emotions, such as hate and resentment, we can create better health, confidence, and emotional fortitude. A member of the spice family, thyme is naturally antimicrobial. It is also a powerful antioxidant and analgesic.

Emotions: Grief, depression, guilt, hatred, resentment, resistance.

Affirmations: Today is a clean slate. I am gentle with myself and others. I am smart and I can find a solution. My intentions are pure.

TURMERIC *(Curcuma longa).*

Turmeric, a perennial plant in the ginger family, has been used for thousands of years in traditional Chinese medicine and other Eastern cultures. The essential oil is steam distilled from the plant's tuberous rhizomes, which boast a beautiful yellow-gold color and a warm, somewhat spicy, and earthy aroma. Pure turmeric oil can be taken internally, diffused, or used aromatically, and has many benefits. Physically, it can support the immune, nervous, and digestive systems. Psychologically, turmeric increases and uplifts the mood to create feelings of positivity and hope. Diffusing the oil promotes mental clarity. Diluting the oil with a carrier oil and massaging into the skin can calm inflammation and nourish the skin.

Emotions: *Depression, discouragement, negativity, hopelessness*

Affirmations: I love and approve of myself. I draw from my inner strength and light. I can find good in bad situations.

VETIVER *(Vetiveria zizanioides).*

Vetiver is tremendously supportive for the multitasking mind that tends to gravitate toward symptoms of ADHD, such as distraction. It helps balance the mind and promotes clarity for those who feel torn between people and priorities, or struggle making simple decisions. Vetiver smells like the earth, and grounds individuals, helping them connect to their true selves. It encourages confidence to know what to do when, and why. It may be used to help restore a healthy sleep cycle, to support focus and attention during the day, and to release painful past trauma in the way of mental focus.

Emotions: *Mental fatigue, resentment, distraction, frustration, anger, trauma, stress, shock, depression, anxiety.*

Affirmations: *I share my opinions freely and easily shrug it off when someone disagrees. I commit to being honest about who I am and what I love. Making wise decisions is easy for me. My life improves every day and in every way because of my wise decisions.*

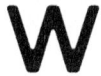

WILD ORANGE *(Citrus sinensis).*
Wild orange is richly mood uplifting and encourages happiness, good health, and a lifetime of joy. It is a powerful essential oil to increase abundance in every area of life. Wild orange brings joy and rids the mind of fear and anxiety. It reminds the soul of innate, universal bliss. Combine wild orange with frankincense daily to support recovery from symptoms of depression. Use the two aromatically and topically for emotional clarity and daily joy.

Emotions: *Depression, grief, irritability, fear, self-criticism, trauma.*

Affirmations: Creative energy surges through me and leads me to new and brilliant ideas. I release struggle and resistance. I am resilient and resourceful. I choose to see how every situation serves me.

WINTERGREEN *(Gaultheria fragrantissima).*

Wintergreen is a natural painkiller. Physically, it can assist with headaches, joint pain, and tissue pain. It also relieves the emotional pain of those who inhale it. Wintergreen teaches us that we do not always need to be right. We can let go of the ways in which we hurt if we're carrying burdens of wrongdoing by others. It can help us release the pain associated with our own trials. It also teaches us that we do not need to carry burdens alone.

Emotions: Anger, stress, aggravation, grief, guilt,overwhelm.

Affirmations: I am open to the possibility of peace. I feel centered in the peaceful, loving energy of my heart. I can release my past and live calmly and serenely. No matter what events occur during the day, I remain calm and centered. I am open to receiving support. I bring peace into moments of chaos.

Y

YLANG YLANG *(Cananga odorata).*

Ylang ylang helps us open our hearts and restore the child within us. It is physically useful for heart conditions. Ylang ylang suggests to our minds and hearts that we can open to feel love, joy, and emotional safety. Consequently, ylang ylang can assist people who have gone through intense emotional traumas, helping them to let go of the pain and move forward in life.

Emotions: *Trauma, resistance, numbness, discouragement, fear.*

Affirmations: *I live bravely and boldly. I choose to see myself as whole and unbroken. My heart leads me to experience the best in life. Like the depths of the ocean, my mind is calm in each moment.*

ESSENTIAL OIL BLENDS

The list of oil blends that follow is organized from A to Z by purpose. (For example, relaxation or anti-aging.) Accompanying each entry is general information about the oil blend, such as the oils it may contain, and emotional states it may benefit.

Note: Oil blends may be used aromatically, topically, and/or internally (only when it is specified that it is safe to do so on the product labels on their packaging). Many blends require dilution with a carrier oil, such as almond oil, coconut oil, grapeseed oil, or jojoba oil, if they are to be applied directly on the skin.

A

ALIGNING BLEND™
(bergamot, coriander, marjoram, peppermint, jasmine, rose)
Ancient Egyptians called coriander the "spice of happiness." As such, it is the perfect oil to combine with uplifting bergamot and calming marjoram to form the primary components of this powerful aligning blend. Smaller amounts of peppermint, jasmine, and rose essential oils, mixed with fractionated coconut oil, round out the blend. This special combination promotes harmony and progression in our lives and encourages us to explore new possibilities while we stay centered and grounded.

ANCHORING BLEND™
(lavender, cedarwood, frankincense, sandalwood, cinnamon, black pepper, patchouli)
The primary oils in this blend—lavender, cedarwood, and frankincense—are enhanced with sandalwood, cinnamon, black pepper, and patchouli in a base of fractionated coconut oil to create a stabilizing oil that calms and soothes the nervous system, allowing you to connect with your authentic self. It can bring clarity of mind when your thoughts are scattered and you feel unhinged or alone. It restores trust in self as it powerfully anchors you to the present and restores feelings of completeness. It is a valuable oil to diffuse or apply during meditation or yoga because it encourages the release of negative energy and grounds you to the task at hand.

ANTI-AGING BLEND
(frankincense, sandalwood, lavender, myrrh)
This blend of essential oils encourages spiritual wellbeing and growth. It encourages hope, faith, and gratitude while ridding the body and soul of consuming darkness. It helps us to be present at the moment and understand our spirits and the role of divine power in our lives. Also, it's useful for the treatment of skin blemishes and wrinkles.

ARISING BLEND™
(grapefruit, lemon, osmanthus, melissa, siberian fir)
Wonderfully fragrant and bursting with energy, this oil is a delightful blend of grapefruit, lemon, osmanthus, Melissa, and Siberian fir in a base of fractionated coconut oil. The energizing properties of grapefruit and lemon pair beautifully with the calming and uplifting alpha-pinene, beta-pinene, and bornyl acetate compounds in Siberian fir. The floral tones in osmanthus and Melissa boost the blend's refreshing aroma, while the soothing power of frankincense makes the oil a perfect blend to apply topically. Whether it is inhaled, diffused, or massaged into the skin, this blend promotes freedom, enlightenment, and inspiration.

BRAVE BLEND™
(wild orange, amyris, osmanthus, cinnamon bark)
This bright, warm blend is energizing and vibrant, making it

perfect for those moments in life that require courage: facing a new day, starting a new job, tackling a big project, working through bumps in relationships, processing change, and so many others. The oils chosen for the blend—wild orange, amyris, osmanthus, and cinnamon—are ideal tools for mustering courage and confidence. Wild orange is energizing and cleansing. Amyris soothes anxiety. Osmanthus, sourced from the flowers of the Osmanthus fragrans plant native to China, carries a subtle hint of apricot or peaches and is used in Eastern medicine for a variety of health purposes. It is used here as a mood lifter. Cinnamon is uplifting and comforting. Roll over the back of the neck and your pulse points to banish doubt. Apply to the wrists and inhale when you're feeling unmotivated. Roll on the bottoms of the feet to encourage positivity and foster courage.

C

CALMER BLEND™
(lavender, cananga, buddha wood, roman chamomile)
This sweet, woody, and relaxing blend draws on the power of lavender, cananga, Buddha wood, and Roman chamomile essential oils to reduce tension, promote rest, and wipe out worries. It is particularly helpful at bed time when rolled on the bottoms of the feet, smoothed over the back of the neck, or applied to the wrists and inhaled. Each of the oils selected for this blend have highly soothing properties. Two of them may not be familiar but have much in common with the more well-known oils lavender and Roman chamomile.

Cananga is a plant in the same family as the cananga tree (Cananga odorata), from which ylang ylang is extracted. Like ylang ylang and other floral oils, cananga oil is known to help reduce stress. Its warm, beautiful scent creates a relaxing and inviting environment at bedtime. Buddha wood essential oil comes from the Eremophila mitchellii plant, which is commonly known as false sandalwood and is native to Australia.The oil is often used for meditation because it is both grounding and soothing.

CALMING BLEND
(lavender, marjoram, Roman chamomile, ylang ylang)
This blend of essential oils helps heal the heart and encourages us to forgive by reducing the impact of emotions such as hate, anger, fear, and resentment. As these emotions fade, we can feel more compassion for others and accept that no one is perfect.

CELLULAR REPAIR BLEND
(frankincense, wild orange, lemongrass, thyme, summer savory)
This blend repairs emotional patterns that are found in our DNA. It encourages individuals who feel they are stuck in those destructive patterns to see the light of a new day. It helps to shift the energy in the body and reminds us that we can change and life will get better. This blend works well for any mental health condition.

CLEANSING BLEND
(lemon, lime, pine, citronella)
This powerful essential oil blend helps individuals who feel burdened by the toxicity of destructive habits and patterns. It cleanses the soul of heavy emotions, thereby providing space for emotional breakthroughs.

COMFORTING BLEND
(frankincense, patchouli, ylang ylang, labdanum, amyris, sandalwood, rose, osmanthus)
This blend helps soothe feelings of sadness and depression. If we are grieving the death of a loved one, it may ease the pain of our loss. It reminds us that we are whole in the part of us that is not bound to the body. The oils in this blend promote balance in the hormonal system, creating overall wellbeing.

D

DETOXIFICATION BLEND
(clove, grapefruit, thyme, and geranium)
This blend helps us cleanse our organs. It reduces the effect of harmful environmental toxins and microbes that enter our bodies. Emotionally, it also aids us when we are going through changes and transitions.

DIGESTIVE BLEND
(ginger, peppermint, tarragon, fennel, caraway)
This blend is for those who struggle to digest the process of life, and thus, may feel overwhelmed and exhausted. It helps individuals see how to accomplish tasks one at a time, in a digestible fashion. It can cleanse the gut and by doing so, reestablish motivation by helping the brain receive peace and clearer instruction.

E

ENCOURAGING BLEND
(peppermint, clementine, coriander, basil, yuzu, Melissa, rosemary)

In times of emotional uncertainty, this oil gives us the courage we need to follow the path ahead of us. It reminds us of our own goodness and releases us from stress that comes from the negative belief that we "are not good enough." For those who are anxious about meeting a specific challenge, such as taking an important test or breaking bad news, it can calm the nerves and help with focus.

F

FEMININE CELEBRATION BLEND
(patchouli, bergamot, sandalwood, rose, jasmine, cinnamon, cistus, vetiver, ylang ylang)

This blend celebrates feminine nature and supports female energy and body function. It helps to calm feelings of tension, reduce unhealthy pride and competitiveness, and can encourage positive nurturing and adaptability. It also can help a broken motherchild relationship. This blend is particularly helpful for helping women connect to their feminine side.

FOCUS BLEND
(amyris, patchouli, frankincense, lime, ylang ylang)
This blend is used to help individuals who have a hard time staying focus and finishing the task at hand. It is an excellent choice for those with ADHD symptoms or who work in a distracting environment, such as a shared office. The focus blend calms and grounds the mind, causing us to stay present and finish what is in front of us.

G

GROUNDING BLEND
(spruce, ho wood, frankincense, blue tansy, blue chamomile)
This blend is composed entirely of tree oils. Think of a tree rooting itself deep into the ground so it may grow tall and live long. Essential oils in the tree family remind us to be firmly rooted. When this blend is applied topically, it encourages us to reconnect to our roots and learn patience when trying to achieve goals. It teaches us to see the bigger perspective, find inner strength, and reestablish our lives in ways that help us grow tall and strong. This blend can help with jetlag, symptoms of depression, and headaches.

H

HEADACHE RELIEF BLEND.
(See Tension blend).

I

INSECT REPELLENT BLEND
(lemon, eucalyptus, citronella)
This oil blend is a wonderful way to keep bugs away—
including that which "bugs" us in life. Thus, it may serve as
an emotional shield. Those who tend to hold others burdens
and negative emotions will benefit from this blend. It helps
us create emotional boundaries so we don't absorb and
carry feelings that aren't ours.

INSPIRING BLEND
*(cardamom, cinnamon, ginger, clove, sandalwood,
jasmine, damiana)*
This powerful blend helps to restore our passion for life and
helps instill us with the courage to pursue our dreams. It
promotes enthusiasm and affection. Those who are working
to achieve a great and important purpose will feel refreshed
by its scent.

INVIGORATING BLEND
(wild orange, lemon, grapefruit, mandarin, bergamot, tangerine)

All citrus essential oils are natural mood lifters. They naturally trigger a good mood, mental clarity, and feelings of peace and happiness. When blended together, these essential oils can support creativity of mind and a burst of joy, energy, and inner peace. Everyone has the right to create. This blend helps us imagine and have confidence in our creations. Through using the creative part of the brain, we then feel the spark of life again. This blend can encourage happiness when diffused and is an excellent daily blend to diffuse at home or at the office.

J

JOYFUL BLEND
(lavandin, tangerine, elemi, lemon myrtle, Melissa, ylang ylang)

This blend is for individuals who are depressed. It cleanses energy and calms the heart. It makes the heart more open to relaxation, joy, courage, and light by encouraging us to reach our goals. It may teach us that fear and worry don't need to take us down and we can get what we want in life. This blend is particularly helpful for emotional imbalance that may surface with symptoms of depression.

M

MASSAGE BLEND
(basil, grapefruit, cypress, marjoram)
This blend is used to help the mind and body relax. It helps ease tension in the body. It also helps to soothe the souls of people who are going through sorrow or feel overwhelmed with stress. By helping them relax and let go on a deep level, energy can start freely moving again through their bodies. This helps people move forward in life peacefully.

METABOLIC BLEND
(grapefruit, lemon, peppermint, and ginger)
This essential oil is for individuals who struggle with loving their bodies. It encourages self-worth and helps release negative emotions about body image. It seeks to regulate metabolism, and in doing so, may regulate emotions that prevent healthy digestion of the life's natural ebbs and flows. As we work through issues related to body image and metabolizing life, we may learn to love our and honor our human body and appreciate the miracle and blessing that it is for us.

P

PROTECTIVE BLEND
(wild orange, clove, cinnamon)
This blend helps strengthen the immunity and provides us with physical protection from viruses and harmful bacteria. Emotionally, this blend protects us by strengthening our inner selves, encouraging us to stand up for what we believe. It helps us to create boundaries and not let harmful energy around us into our personal energy field where it may deplete us.

R

REASSURING BLEND
(vetiver, lavender, ylang ylang, frankincense, clary sage, marjoram, labdanum, spearmint)
This blend is appropriate for times of worry when negative thoughts are swirling in the mind and we just can't let them go. Those who tend to obsess about their plans, at the expense of being present in the now, may find this blend helps them to relax and find more contentment at the moment.

RENEWING BLEND
(spruce, bergamot, juniper berry, myrrh, arborvitae, nootka tree, thyme, citronella)

If we are troubled by past decisions or feel guilty and ashamed about our choices or actions, this blend can help us forgive ourselves and find a resolution. It takes a weight off the mind and soothes the heart. Renewal of the spirit often comes during moments of prayer, meditation, or contemplation—and this oil blend enhances those experiences elevating and grounding simultaneously.

RESCUER BLEND™
(copaiba, lavender, spearmint, zanthoxylum)

This soothing blend is ideal for anyone who regularly participates in intense activity or experiences tension in the shoulders, legs, or back. Composed of copaiba, lavender, spearmint, and zanthoxylum essential oils, the blend can be rolled over tired shoulders, achy legs, and worn out feet. As it soothes muscles and skin, it also calms the mind and refreshes the senses. Its aroma is woody, minty, and floral all at once and provides just the rescue you need after a long day of activity. The spearmint in the blend lifts the mood and helps restore energy. The lavender and copaiba help reduce stress in the muscles and in the mind. The lesser-known zanthoxylum essential oil is steam distilled from the dried berries of Zanthoxylum armatum, or winged prickly ash trees. Its fruity and alluring scent blends beautifully with the other oils in the blend, and it adds an extra layer of soothing and uplifting properties.

RESPIRATORY BLEND
(laurel leaf, peppermint, eucalyptus, melaleuca)

This oil blend supports a healthy life through breathing and releasing grief and pain that may be taking the breath right out of us. As we take a breath in and out each day, we have the opportunity to let go and allow new life and possibilities to enter our mind and body. This blend encourages us to do just that--to balance our life by breathing out what hurts and breathing in encouragement, light, and hope for a restful and joyful future. Physically, this blend is helpful for respiratory issues and can support healthy breathing.

RESTFUL BLEND
(lavender, cedarwood, ho wood, ylang ylang, marjoram, Roman chamomile, vetiver, Hawaiian sandalwood)
This blend addresses the emotional states that can interfere with sleep. Whether it is stress, excitement, or anxiety that keeps us from letting go of the day or staying asleep in the middle of the night, this oil blend is a companion we can trust to help us feel calm so we may rest.

S

SKIN-CLEARING BLEND
(black cumin seed, rosewood, melaleuca, eucalyptus)
This blend has very positive properties that help with skin health. Emotionally, it helps individuals that have suppressed emotions (such as anger and guilt) reduce a tendency to lash out at people. This blend encourages self-acceptance and healthy release of negative emotions. It's particularly helpful for relieving feelings of aggravation, self-hate, or self-rejection that may surface through the skin as acne.

SOOTHING BLEND
(wintergreen, camphor, peppermint, blue tansy, blue chamomile)
This blend helps release emotional issues that may be causing physical pain. By bringing struggle and agony to the surface, it can be released and consequently, may relieve the physical body of pain and trauma. Consequently, this blend is helpful for physical pain management.

STEADY BLEND™
(amyris, balsam fir, coriander, magnolia)
This grounding blend of amyris, balsam fir, coriander, and magnolia essential oils is an ideal mood balancer. It relaxes the mind while also helping you feel rooted and grounded in the present. Amyris essential oil is steam distilled from the dried bark of Amryis baslamifera, commonly referred to as Indian sandalwood and originating from the West Indies. Its scent, however, is quite unlike sandalwood oil and carries very subtle undertones of vanilla. Amyris is a valuable tool in relieving anxiety and pairs well with the other aromatic oils in this blend. Like amryis, balsam fir is a warm, woody oil and is often used to relieve stress. Coriander and magnolia each promote relaxation and round out the blend. Rolling the blend over the bottoms of the feet will steady your emotions throughout the day. Applying to the temples or the wrists can help reduce anxiety.

STRONGER BLEND™
(cedarwood, litsea, frankincense, rose)
This blend of precious rose, frankincense, litsea, and cedarwood essential oils protects and heals skin but can also protect the mind from negative emotions that crop up in stressful situations. Its scent is lemony, bright, and slightly herbal. Each of the oils in the blend is known for having restorative properties that soothe irritated skin and clear imperfections. These oils also work wonders on the

mind, promoting renewal and resilience. The blend is great for rolling over knees, feet, and hands after an active day outdoors. Smoothing it over skin irritations and blemishes will calm the skin and promote healing. Applying it to the temples and wrists when you need to feel strong and resilient will draw confidence from within.

T

TENSION BLEND
(wintergreen, lavender, peppermint, frankincense, cilantro, Roman chamomile, marjoram)
Also known as the headache relief blend, this blend helps individuals who are emotionally overwhelmed to let go of the stress that may be causing tension in the body. It helps to calm and relax the mind so that tension can be resolved and released. This blend is particularly helpful for treatment of headaches and migraines associated with fear, anger, frustration, resentment, and other forms of emotional upset.

THINKER BLEND™
(vetiver, peppermint, clementine, rosemary)
This bright and earthy blend of vetiver, peppermint, clementine, and rosemary oils is ideal for bringing details into focus, blocking out noise, and working creatively. It can be used every day to promote clarity, impart energy, and reduce mental distractions. Each of the oils in this blend plays a unique role in supporting concentration and

bringing positivity to challenging tasks. Clementine boosts the mood, while peppermint works to improve cognition and fight fatigue. Vetiver calms worried minds and combats anxious thoughts, and rosemary is energizing while also promoting feelings of being grounded and capable. The blend can be rolled over the wrists and temples or simply inhaled straight from the bottle. And because it is safe and natural, it can be reapplied as needed during long periods of concentration.

U

UPLIFTING BLEND
(wild orange, clove, star anise, lemon myrtle, nutmeg, cinnamon)
When we need to cheer up or promote positivity in a particular environment, this may be the blend of choice. Highly distressed people may find that it helps heal their hearts. Those who are down in the dumps or just feel sluggish and disengaged may find that it spices things up for them and restores their enthusiasm for living.

WOMEN'S MONTHLY BLEND
(clary sage, lavender, bergamot, Roman chamomile, cedarwood, ylang ylang, geranium, fennel, carrot seed)

This essential oil blend supports healthy relationships. It teaches us to be open and vulnerable at times so that we may rid ourselves of the fear of rejection. It helps us maintain emotional balance within our life by teaching us to safely accept the ideas, thoughts, and feelings of others who love us. In turn, it helps us to feel the love in our relationships. It's useful for addressing emotions related to women's monthly cycles.

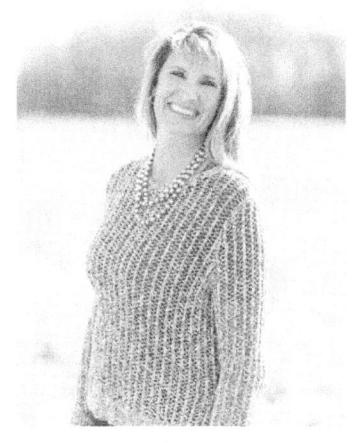

ABOUT THE AUTHOR

Rebecca Linder Hintze, M.Sc., is a family issues expert, former broadcast journalist, and bestselling author of Healing Your Family History (Hay House, 2006), which has been translated into eight languages; Essentially Happy (Visium Group, 2014); and Essential Oils for Happy Living (Visium Group, 2017). She holds a bachelor's degree from Brigham Young University and a master of science degree from the University of East London, School of Psychology. A mother of four grown children, she currently resides in Northern Virginia with her husband, Shane.

Printed in Great Britain
by Amazon